The Master's Touch

AIDS

A Christian Perspective

By Howard E. Mueller
Edited by Roger Sonnenberg
and Thomas J. Doyle

CPH
SAINT LOUIS

Assistant to the editor: Cynthia Anderson

3558 South Jefferson Avenue, St. Louis, MO 63118-3968
Manufactured in the United States of America

1 2 3 4 5 6 7 8 9 10 05 04 03 02 01 00 99 98 97 96

Contents

1

AIDS—Its Challenge

Focusing Our Sights

In this session we will see that AIDS is a fatal virus-borne disease that spreads a pall of fear and grief over people. Despite the tragedy of AIDS, the disease offers God's people an opportunity to show the world God's love and compassion offered freely through faith in Christ Jesus.

Focusing Our Attention

A Mother's Diary—Entry 1

(This diary is a composite of typical experiences.)

Last Friday, Peter called, said he was terribly sick with AIDS and asked if he could come home. I covered the mouthpiece, asked Wes (my husband) and then said a hesitant yes. Today Peter came home, thin, haggard, and obviously sick. He is 32, but he looks like an old man. His voice is thin, his manner uncertain. This is my son Peter—a stranger. Wes said hello and little more.

I'm scared. Taking care of him—touching him—will I get AIDS? He's been in the hospital with a rare pneumonia several times. It seems so weird, so unreal: Peter is going to die! He'll never get married or have children. In Peter's actions, I see Death walking around our lives.

Before he left home eight years ago, I wondered why he hadn't shown an interest in girls. Is he homosexual? Whatever the case, his "alternate" lifestyle suddenly seems to fill our house.

My world is crashing in around me. Will Wes and Peter start talking to one another and get on better terms? It's clear to me that our lives will revolve around Peter until ... Peter has become the center of my life again—a grown man yet my little boy again. Even as I look outside, homes in the neighborhood—and the people in them—seem strangely far away. Will we have the strength to see this through? O God, what's happened to us?

Our pastor called yesterday, not his usual self. He seemed distant—afraid? Conversation with Peter was strained. It was like two actors reading their lines for the first time. Before he left, pastor asked to wash his hands. I gave him a fresh towel. Wes told him, "Pastor, people won't take it well if they know you're visiting here. We'll be all right." O God, help us through this.

Focusing on the Issue

A million Americans—1 in every 250—are infected with HIV. Within 10 years the majority of those infected with HIV will develop AIDS. This means that most people within their lifetime will know some person—a friend, relative, or acquaintance—who is HIV or AIDS affected.

1. Peter has come home with AIDS. Describe some of the ways his illness will affect his family and his community.

2. The presence of AIDS often divides people. How might the disease bring them closer together?

3. What responsibility, if any, does the Christian community have to Peter and his family? Should the pastor call on Peter and his family despite the fact that he might be criticized by other church members?

4. Is a Christian obligated to take on personal risk in order to care for someone with a deadly transmissible disease? Read Mark 1:40–42. What is the risk of contracting AIDS in casual personal contact?

A man with leprosy came to Him and begged Him on his knees, "If You are willing, You can make me clean."

Filled with compassion, Jesus reached out His hand and touched the man. "I am willing," He said. "Be clean!" Immediately the leprosy left him and he was cured. (Mark 1:40–42)

Focusing on God's Word

1. Underline those words or phrases in 1 Corinthians 12:12–27 that speak to the church about Peter and his family.

The body is a unit, though it is made up of many parts; and though all its parts are many, they form one body. So it is with Christ. For we were all baptized by one Spirit into one body—whether Jews or Greeks, slave or free—and we were all given the one Spirit to drink.

Now the body is not made up of one part but of many. If the foot should say, "Because I am not a hand, I do not belong to the body," it would not for that reasons cease to be part of the body. And if the ear should say, "Because I am not an eye, I do not belong to the body," it would not for that reason cease to be part of the body. If the whole body were an eye, where would the sense of hearing be? If the whole body were an ear, where would the sense of smell be? But in fact God has arranged the parts in the body, every one of them, just as He wanted them to be. If they were all one part, where would the body be? As it is, there are many parts, but one body.

The eye cannot say to the hand, "I don't need you!" And the head cannot say to the feet, "I don't need you!" On the contrary, those parts of the body that seem to be weaker are indispensable, and the parts that we think are less honorable we treat with special honor. And the parts that are unpresentable are treated with special modesty, while our presentable parts need no special treatment. But God has combined the members of the body and has given greater honor to the parts that lacked it, so that there would be no division in the body, but that its parts should have equal concern for each other. If one part suffers, every part suffers with it; if one part is honored, every part rejoices with it.

Now you are the body of Christ, and each one of you is a part of it. (1 Corinthians 12:12–27)

a. Describe the church according to St. Paul with Peter and his family as a part of that church.

b. Do you think it's fair that the entire membership suffer if another's suffering is due to his or her sinfulness (v. 26)?

c. Do you think it's fair that one should die or be punished for the sins of another? Why?

2. Review Matthew 25:31, 34–40. Underline each word that might describe Barbara's family (e.g., "sick"). After doing so, share with a partner why you underlined the words or phrases that you did. Discuss with the entire class how the Christian community can meet the Lord's expectations with reference to this family.

"When the Son of Man comes in His glory, and all the angels with Him, He will sit on His throne in heavenly glory. ... Then the King will say to those on His right, 'Come, you who are blessed by My Father; take your inheritance, the kingdom prepared for you since the creation of the world. For I was hungry and you gave Me something to eat, I was thirsty and you gave Me something to drink, I was a stranger and you invited Me in, I needed clothes and you clothed Me, I was sick and you looked after Me, I was in prison and you came to visit Me.'

"Then the righteous will answer Him, 'Lord, when did we see You hungry and feed You, or thirsty and give You something to drink? When did we see You a stranger and invite You in, or needing clothes and clothe You? When did we see You sick or in prison and go to visit You?'

"The King will reply, 'I tell you the truth, whatever you did for one of the least of these brothers of Mine, you did for Me.' " (Matthew 25:31, 34–40)

3. (a) In what sense can each of the terms *stranger, sick,* and *prison* apply to Barbara's family?

b. How does the picture of the church as a body and Christ as its head give special meaning to Matthew 25:40?

4. What does Mark 1:40–42 tell us about personal risk in showing compassion to others?

5. *The body of Christ has AIDS*. Why is this statement correct in a spiritual sense of the word? Despite our spiritual AIDS, what is the healing that Jesus Christ provided for us according to Romans 5:18–19?

> Consequently, just as the result of one trespass was condemnation for all men, so also the result of one act of righteousness was justification that brings life for all men. For just as through the disobedience of the one man the many were made sinners, so also through the obedience of the one man the many will be made righteous. (Romans 5:18–19)

6. What promise does God give to Peter and all who suffer from this deadly disease because of their sinful behavior? See 1 John 1:9.

Focusing on My Life

1. Imagine you are Peter's father or mother. How would you react

a. to your son's illness?

b. to Peter wanting to move back home to die?

c. to the people in your congregation who criticized your pastor for visiting Peter?

2. Which of the following things would frighten you the most about the disease? Why?

a. What other people might think.

b. The inconvenience of having a dying person in your house.

c. Acquiring the disease yourself from treating Peter.

Since HIV is in the semen, vaginal secretions, or the blood of an affected person, there are four main ways of spreading HIV: (1) receiving a blood transfusion from an infected person; (2) through sex with an infected person; (3) using contaminated needles to inject drugs; (4) being born from a mother who has HIV.

3. Today's church member has been

described as a consumer, taking from rather than giving to the church. Which attitude best describes yourself? Which attitude best describes the majority of the members of your church?

4. As you are motivated by God's love for you in Jesus, how might you individually or collectively as a congregation enable Peter and his family to be consumers of God's grace and mercy? List specific things you might do to demonstrate God's love in Christ Jesus. How might these things you do and say benefit not only Peter and his family but others in your community in need of God's love for them in Christ?

Focusing on the Week Ahead

Spend some time this week studying information from your local public library about the HIV virus and AIDS. How might you use some of this information to better equip people in your congregation in dealing with the disease?

2

AIDS— Judgment or Grace?

Focusing Our Sights

In this session we will examine the condemnation and judgment that often accompanies the disease of AIDS. We will also see how in contrast, though God hates the sin that often brings about the disease (homosexuality, sexual promiscuity, drug use), He forgives and loves the sinner. This is evident because God willingly gave up His Son Jesus Christ to win forgiveness and eternal life for *all* people.

Focusing Our Attention

A Mother's Diary—Entry 2

"Live" in Wes and Barbara's home as you slowly read the entry in Barbara's diary, noting especially what it says about Peter.

Peter's been home five weeks now—how strange that I'm figuring time from the day he came home. At first, I crash-landed, bewildered and afraid; now I have a better idea what this is about. Peter tries to be as little trouble as possible. He's mature, courteous—and troubled.

What bothers him? He doesn't talk about it. I don't know, and I'm afraid to ask.

When Peter came home, a lifestyle walked in with him that our neighbors and church frown upon. I feel so shamed by all this that I, a people person, can't bring myself to call anyone. The telephone has been silent; I suppose the word has gotten around.

Will Wes and Peter ever be father and son again? Wes, always a man's man, was pretty hard on Peter. Try as he might, Peter felt he always fell short of his father's expectations. Obviously, Wes is terribly disappointed. Can the wounds be healed?

Focusing on the Issue

1. In what way(s) is Peter's return a bittersweet experience?

2. "Do not judge, and you will not be judged" (Luke 6:37). If we do not judge Peter, are we not giving silent consent to his sinful past?

3. "Love does not jeopardize repentance; love calls for repentance." Why is this statement important to remember as we encounter the Peters in our lives?

4. "True acceptance—defined as believing in a person's worth, dignity, and potential—is received as emotional support, not as moral sanction." Why is this statement important for us to remember?

5. In what way can Peter come to life—even while dying—through caring ministry?

Focusing on God's Word

Read John 9:1–5.

As He went along, He saw a man blind from birth. His disciples asked Him, "Rabbi, who sinned, this man or his parents, that he was born blind?" "Neither this man nor his parents sinned," said Jesus, "but this happened so that the work of God might be displayed in his life. As long as it is day, we must do the work of Him who sent Me. Night is coming, when no one can work. While I am in the world, I am the light of the world." (John 9:1–5)

1. (a) Is AIDS, blindness, or any other ailment necessarily a result of one particular person's sin?

b. The argument may be this: Illness is a punishment for sin. Peter is fatally sick with AIDS. Therefore, Peter's illness is God's judgment. How does Jesus destroy this reasoning?

c. If Peter did contract AIDS through homosexual activity, was AIDS a punishment for his sin? or a result of the sinful behavior? or both?

d. In what ways might God use Peter's illness so that the work of God might be displayed in Peter's life? the life of Peter's parents? the lives of the people in his parents' congregation?

Review the picture given to us in Luke 15:11–24 of God and those who get AIDS through sinful sexual activity or drug use.

Jesus continued: "There was a man who had two sons. The younger one said to his father, 'Father, give me my share of the estate.' So he divided his property between them. Not long after that, the younger son got together all he had, set off for a distant country and there squandered his wealth in wild living. After he had spent everything, there was a severe famine in that whole country, and he began to be in need. So he went and hired himself out to a citizen of that country, who sent him to his fields to feed pigs. He longed to fill his stomach with the pods that the pigs were eating, but no one gave him anything. When he came to his senses, he said, 'How many of my father's hired men have food to spare, and here I am starving to death! I will set out and go back to my father and say to him: Father, I have sinned against heaven and against you. I am no longer worthy to be called your son; make me like one of your hired men.' So he got up and went to his father.

"But while he was still a long way off, his father saw him and was filled with compassion for him; he ran to his son, threw his arms around him and kissed him. The son said to him, 'Father, I have sinned against heaven and against you. I am no longer worthy to be called your son.'

"But the father said to his servants, 'Quick! Bring the best robe and put it on him. Put a ring on his finger and sandals on his feet. Bring the fattened calf and kill it. Let's have a feast and celebrate. For this son of mine was dead and is alive again; he was lost and is found.' So they began to celebrate." (Luke 15:11–24)

2. Think about the father in the parable.

a. Should the father be faulted for not trying to stop his son from running off with his inheritance (v. 12)? Why or why not?

b. Should the father be faulted for his silence about his son's sinful past upon the son's return (v. 20)? Why or why not?

c. Should the father make the son pay for his sinful past as opposed to celebrating his return (v. 23)? Why or why not?

3. Think about the son in the parable.

a. Didn't the son get what he deserved when he ended up feeding pigs (v. 15)? Why or why not?

b. Did the son really deserve his father's love and forgiveness (v. 20)? Why or why not?

Read Luke 15:1–2.

> Now the tax collectors and "sinners" were all gathering around to hear Him. But the Pharisees and the teachers of the law muttered, "This man welcomes sinners and eats with them." (Luke 15:1–2)

4. What do these words say about Jesus' love for sinners? for Peter?

Read Matthew 9:12.

> On hearing this, Jesus said, "It is not the healthy who need a doctor, but the sick." (Matthew 9:12)

5. Underline what Jesus did because of His love for sinners and desire to treat their sickness. Circle the words that describe what God has commissioned us to do, including for people who are dying of AIDS.

> Therefore, if anyone is in Christ, he is a new creation; the old has gone, the new has come! All this is from God, who reconciled us to Himself through Christ and gave us the ministry of reconciliation: that God was reconciling the world to Himself in Christ, not counting men's sins against them. And He has committed to us the message of reconciliation (2 Corinthians 5:17–20).

Focusing on My Life

1. As Peter stands before you in your mind, which thought comes first, judgment or love? Why?

2. Which of the following statements do you think are correct when it comes to offering forgiveness to any sinner:

a. Forgiveness means tolerance of sin.
b. Forgiveness means leniency with sin.
c. Forgiveness is always tied to justice.
d. Forgiveness is an empathic, felt event.

3. Which attitude(s) of yours have changed toward people with AIDS as a result of this study? As you are motivated by God's love for you, what attitude will you strive for?

4. Peter has been lost to the Christian community for eight years. Now he is home. Compare the response of the Christian community to the father's response in the parable of the lost son. Then compare their response to the response of the older son in the same parable. See Luke 15:25–31.

Focusing on the Week Ahead

Spend some special time in meditation and prayer in the next week, reading passages such as Matthew 18:21–35 and 1 John 4:7–13. Ask that God would help you be less judgmental and more loving in ministering to anyone who might be infected with the HIV virus or with AIDS.

3

AIDS—The Disease That Isolates

Focusing Our Sights

In this session we will discuss how those directly touched by AIDS often feel isolated from friends, the church, and the neighborhood. Some even feel isolated from God. We can rejoice, however, in the Good News that through His life, death, and resurrection, Jesus Christ destroyed the wall of isolation that separates us from God and other people.

Focusing Our Attention

A Mother's Diary—Entries 3 and 4

Put yourself into Wes and Barbara's situation as you read diary entries 3 and 4. What kind of isolation are you beginning to feel?

Entry 3

I feel so alone—so abandoned. Marsha has called just once. We've always been able to visit by phone. This time our conversation quickly ran out. We've received two cards—both get-

well cards for someone who won't get well. How ironic that between "get well" and "sympathy," card makers have nothing to say!

I feel like I'm always in the presence of this disease, and it's destroying me. I never realized how much I need other people. This terrible disease has walled me off from the people I need.

On Tuesday our parish nurse called. She had called me once before. Again, I told her we were okay. Why? This time she insisted, "We don't want a wall to build up between our congregation and you. Would tomorrow at 2:30 be okay?" I hesitated and agreed. Now I'm both excited and afraid—afraid to let the church see our secret.

Entry 4

Perhaps it will help me think more clearly if I put some of these thoughts on paper. What's happening to me? I used to be so sure of things. Now I'm so confused in my faith. I wasn't like this at all in the past. Sunday school and later my membership classes helped me get clear about my Christian faith, and Jesus the Savior became my good friend. Tell me it's still true. I prayed a lot for Peter after he left. Now I have my answer—a stranger walked through my door, and a deathly sick one at that. He's still troubled, and part of it is religion, I know. Our mealtime prayers are hard for him.

In all this, and being away from church—I haven't been there since that day—I'm getting so confused. If I try to pray, it seems like I'm talking to a stranger, or worse, no one is there.

I feel empty. On Sunday I tried to read the Bible, but the words seemed to be a jumble. Even the Twenty-third Psalm seems to talk to someone else; there seems to be nothing in there for me.

I feel so guilty, as if I carry his guilt because I'm his mother.

Our parish nurse called and said she and her husband would attend the early service next Sunday and come over then to be with Peter so that Wes and I could go to church. I know Peter is safe with her. I know we need to go. I never realized how hard it might be to go to church. We'll see.

Focusing on the Issue

1. Barbara has always been a "people person," and yet now she feels different. From whom is she feeling isolated? Why?

2. In her diary, Barbara tells us that she needs to talk to and connect with people. But what kind of polarization is she feeling between her family and church? Do you think some of the polarization she's feeling is self-imposed? If so, why?

3. Why do you think Barbara is feeling alienated from God?

Focusing on God's Word

1. Compare Genesis 2:18, 20–24 with Genesis 3:6–7 .

The LORD God said, "It is not good for man to be alone. I will make a helper suitable for him." ... But for Adam no suitable helper was found. So the LORD God caused the man to fall into a deep sleep; and while he was sleeping, He took one of the man's ribs and closed up the place with flesh. Then the LORD God made a woman from the rib He had taken out of the man, and He brought her to the man. The man said, "This is now bone of my bones and flesh of my flesh; she shall be called 'woman,' for she was taken out of man." For this reason a man will leave his father and mother and be united to his wife, and they will become one flesh. (Genesis 2:18, 20–24)

When the woman saw that the fruit of the tree was good for food and pleasing to the eye, and also desirable for gaining wisdom, she took some and ate it. She also gave some to her husband, who was with her, and he ate it. Then the eyes of both of them were opened, and they realized they were naked; so they sewed fig leaves together and made coverings for themselves. (Genesis 3:6–7)

a. Underline the evidence that God created people to be social beings, people connected to people.

b. Identify one immediate result of the separation between God and mankind because of sin (3:7).

c. A loving God could not bear to be separated from His people. Read aloud His solution to the malady of sin.

"For ... we were reconciled to Him through the death of His Son, how much more, having been reconciled, shall we be saved through His life!" (Romans 5:10)

2. Read John 5:1–9.

Some time later, Jesus went up to Jerusalem for a feast of the Jews. Now there is in Jerusalem near the Sheep Gate a pool, which in Aramaic is called Bethesda and which is surrounded by five covered colonnades. Here a great number of disabled people used to lie—the blind, the lame, the paralyzed. One who was there had been an invalid for thirty-eight years. When Jesus saw him lying there and learned that he had been in this condition for a long time, He asked him, "Do you want to get well?"

"Sir," the invalid replied, "I have no one to help me into the pool when the water is stirred. While I am trying to get in, someone else goes down ahead of me."

Then Jesus said to him, "Get up! Pick up your mat and walk." At once the man was cured; he picked up his mat and walked. (John 5:1–9)

a. In what way do the words *I have no one* (v. 7) describe how Barbara feels?

b. Why do you think the invalid may have felt painfully alone even though he was often surrounded by many people waiting for the water to stir in the nearby pool?

c. In what way did Jesus heal the man's isolation as well as his paralysis?

3. Read the words of David in Psalm 13:1–3.

> How long, O LORD? Will You forget me forever? How long will You hide Your face from me?
> How long must I wrestle with my thoughts and every day have sorrow in my heart? How long will my enemy triumph over me?
> Look on me and answer, O LORD my God. Give light to my eyes, or I will sleep in death. (Psalm 13:1–3)

a. What comfort is there in knowing that a man of great faith such as King David felt separated from God?

b. Who is the "enemy" in Barbara's life? Who is her Friend? In what ways can others help Barbara see who her real Friend is? How might others be "Jesus with skin on" to Barbara and her family?

Focusing on My Life

1. Based on your own experience, can you identify with Barbara's isolation? If so, how and when?

2. What does it mean to a Christian community when one of its members experiences brokenness and need?

3. Assume that after the parish nurse has made her call, she comes to your study group, asking for volunteers to visit Barbara, Wes, and Peter. Will you volunteer? Why or why not?

4. Read aloud 1 Corinthians 13:4–7. In what way do St. Paul's words speak to you about the needs of Barbara and others in your own congregation?

> Love is patient, love is kind. It does not envy, it does not boast, it is not proud. It is not rude, it is not self-seeking, it is not easily angered, it keeps no record of wrongs. Love does not delight in evil but rejoices with the truth. It always protects, always trusts, always hopes, always perseveres. (1 Corinthians 13:4–7)

Focusing on the Week Ahead

Just as Barbara felt lonely, so we feel lonely and isolated at times, even from God. Read the following passages from Scripture as a reminder of God's promises in the wake of loneliness: Psalm 23, Psalm 27:10, Psalm 42, Psalm 91:11, Isaiah 41:10, Matthew 28:20, and Hebrews 13:5–6.

4

Healing from God

Focusing Our Sights

In this session we will review how sin keeps healing from happening. However, we can rejoice that God's love for us in Christ Jesus destroyed sin and enables healing to take place in miraculous ways.

Focusing Our Attention

A Mother's Diary—Entries 5 and 6

Read diary entries 5 and 6. Note the difference in Barbara's home in these two entries.

Entry 5

I can't believe it. It's been months since Peter came home. I feel better inside, more connected. Things are better but not with Peter. His health is going downhill. He is weaker, not out of bed as much as before.

Marsha and two other people from church have been visiting. I never realized how much I need people, how empty I was. They're wonderful people. They don't snow me with words. They let me tell them what's been happening here. I feel 10 pounds lighter, getting these things off my chest. It's as if they're walking down my life path with me. I don't know what I'd do without them.

Wes and Peter are getting along better. I usually leave the room so that they can talk father to son and son to father. Now they respect one another and are friends for the first time in years. How did it happen? I'm not sure. I know I've prayed a lot—I can pray again! Going to church has been as good for Wes as for me. Then I think that every month of Peter's remaining life has put the question to him and Wes: How do you want to part, friends or enemies, reconciled or angry?

Our pastor has been coming back. At first, I think, Peter's past lifestyle was in the forefront of his mind, and conversation didn't come easy. But lately, the pastor seems more relaxed. He respects Peter, mentions Peter's gifts and, I hope, sees in Peter the follower of Jesus he has become. The pastor continually reminds Peter that God claimed him as His own in Holy Baptism. Now whenever the pastor comes, I see the picture of the Good Shepherd looking hopefully for his lost sheep. And in another room I pray that he will.

Entry 6

Things have changed a lot, and I don't think they will get better. Peter doesn't have much time left. Yesterday we brought him home from the hospital. Did we do the right thing? This time he almost died. He's terribly weak, just skin and bones. Peter has no fight left—he wants to die. I'm so tired I sometimes wish, too, that it were all over. Then I ask myself what kind of mother I am.

I'm so tired, running to the hospital, seeing my child at death's door, trying to keep up the house, and now every time he coughs, I jump. Every time he calls out, his thin voice a whisper, I come running. I'm so afraid Peter will choke or something, and I won't know what to do or will do the wrong thing. I can't bear that. And, I'm responsible. Right now the most delicious thing in the world would be a two-hour nap. Dream on, Barbara.

Focusing on the Issue

1. Why is Barbara feeling more connected again?

2. What has happened to Barbara and Wes as a result of their returning to that which, through the Holy Spirit, provided faith-strengthening power—God's Word?

3. What effect might the caring offered within Wes and Barbara's Christian community have on the public?

4. How might the Christian community continue to support each member of Barbara's family in Peter's final days?

a. Barbara

b. Wes

c. Peter

Focusing on God's Word

Read Luke 24:13–32.

Now that same day two of them were going to a village called Emmaus, about seven miles from Jerusalem. They were talking with each other about everything that had happened. As they talked and discussed these things with each other, Jesus Himself came up and walked along with them; but they were kept from recognizing Him. He asked them, "What are you discussing together as you walk along?" They stood still, their faces downcast. One of them, named Cleopas, asked Him, "Are you only a visitor to Jerusalem and do not know the things that have happened there in these days?" "What things?" He asked. "About Jesus of Nazareth," they replied. "He was a prophet, powerful in word and deed before God and all the people. The chief priests and our rulers handed Him over be sentenced to death, and they crucified Him; but we had hoped that He was the one who was going to redeem Israel. And what is more, it is the third day since all this took place. In addition, some of our women amazed us. They went to the tomb early this morning but didn't find His body. They came and told us that they had seen a vision of angels, who said He was alive. Then some of our companions went to the tomb and found it just as the women had said, but Him they did not see." He said to them, "How foolish you are, and how slow of heart to believe all that the prophets have spoken! Did not the Christ have to suffer these things and then enter His glory?" And beginning with Moses and all the Prophets, He explained to them what was said in all the Scriptures concerning Himself. As they approached the village to which they were going, Jesus acted as if He were going farther. But they urged Him strongly, "Stay with us, for it is nearly evening; the day is almost over." So He went in to stay with them. When He was at the table with them, He took bread, gave thanks, broke it and began to give it to them. Then their eyes were opened and they recognized Him, and He disappeared from their sight. They asked each other, "Were not our hearts burning within us while He talked with us on the road and opened the Scriptures to us?" (Luke 24:13–32)

1. This passage is an excellent example of caring support through listening.

a. What need(s) do the disciples bound for Emmaus and Barbara have in common?

b. How did Jesus respond to the needs of the disciples?

c. What did Jesus do to assure the disciples as He reviewed the Old Testament prophecies?

d. What evidence is there in the text that proves Jesus was helpful?

2. How does the Resurrection account prove the statement: "God uses for His glory those people and things that are the most perfectly broken?"

Read Psalm 73:16–17, 21–25.

> When I tried to understand all this, it was oppressive to me till I entered the sanctuary of God; then I understood their final destiny. ... When my heart was grieved and my spirit embittered, I was senseless and ignorant; I was a brute beast before You. Yet I am always with You; You hold me by my right hand. You guide me with Your counsel, and afterward You will take me into glory. Whom have I in heaven but You? And earth has nothing I desire besides You. (Psalm 73:16–17, 21–25)

3. Though their problems were quite different, Barbara's and the psalmist's return to the house of God restored their trust and joy in God. As you reflect on the blessings you have received in worship, how did returning to the sanctuary of God help Barbara and Wes? How has it helped you as you have faced difficult times?

Read Colossians 3:13–14.

> Bear with each other and forgive whatever grievances you may have against one another. Forgive as the Lord forgave you. And over all these virtues put on love, which binds them all together in perfect unity. (Colossians 3:13–14)

The message of the Gospel is one of forgiveness through Jesus Christ.

4. Which of the following people needed forgiveness? Why?

a. Wes

b. Barbara

c. Peter

d. The congregation

e. The pastor

Focusing on My Life

1. As you read Barbara's diary entries, which of the following things did you come to better realize?

a. I need to be a better listener.

b. I need to connect better with members who are hurting in our congregation.

c. I need to appreciate more how demanding and difficult it must be for my pastor as he ministers to the needs of people in our congregation.

d. I need to rethink about how prejudiced I am against certain people and their diseases.

e. I need to draw closer to God when I experience pain in my life.

f. I need Christ and His forgiveness constantly.

g. Other ______________________________.

2. Mother Teresa has said of AIDS: "God is speaking to us in this disease." What is He saying?

3. In what way has your appreciation of the importance of the Christian community's support of individuals and families in crisis grown due to the study?

4. Peter died shortly after Barbara wrote her sixth entry. After reading the final entry, answer the questions that follow.

Entry 7

Two months ago today we buried Peter. I feel a terrible sense of loss, and tears may stain this page before I'm through. But I also feel that Peter closed his eyes knowing his mother loved him, his father loved him, and Jesus loved him. I've lived a lifetime these past 10 months. AIDS has aged me. I'm afraid to look into the mirror, but I'm not afraid to look into my heart. There I feel peace with God, with Peter, with Wes, with people, and with myself.

I was afraid of the funeral. Would there be a single spray of flowers and possibly 10 people? Well, I shouldn't have been. There were flowers from my guild and, especially touching, a spray from Peter's confirmation class—those still around. As funeral attendance goes today, the number of people present was good. They came to give us support, and I love them for it. People were so generous in what they said. Even some men with AIDS came and said how well we cared for Peter. I hope we were a witness for Christ to them.

The pastor's sermon was wonderful. He talked about Peter's final steps on his life journey as a wonderful demonstration of the grace of God in a human life. Loving Peter, Jesus moved him to repent. Peter received complete forgiveness for all sins, and a wonderful peace.

How can I thank my church, the people who showed Christ's love and warmth? They turned what started as a nightmare into a triumph for Peter, Wes, and me.

Now it's time to move on, but I will never forget Peter. How can I remember best? I know! By helping others in their struggles.

a. What kind of continuing support does Barbara need after the funeral?

b. What kind of support could you or your congregation offer to those who grieve the loss of a loved one?

Focusing on the Week Ahead

Reflect on how you and your congregation might help those in their struggle with AIDS or any other disease.

For the Leader

1

AIDS—Its Challenge

Focusing Our Sights

(*About 2 Minutes*)

Read aloud and discuss briefly the goals for this session.

Focusing Our Attention

(*About 5 Minutes*)

Ask a volunteer to read aloud the first entry in "A Mother's Diary." Allow a few moments for participants to share their reactions.

Focusing on the Issue

(*About 10 Minutes*)

Read the opening paragraph.

1. Ask participants to brainstorm ways that Peter's illness might affect his family and community.

2. Ask the participants if they think that the presence of AIDS could actually bring a family closer together. Answers will vary.

3. Answers will vary. Some might cite Matthew 25:40: "The King will reply, 'I tell you the truth, whatever you did for one of the least of these brothers of Mine, you did for Me.' " Jesus tells us that as we treat others, so we are treating Him. Possible negative positions might argue that "Peter made his bed, now he has to lie in it." They might also claim that if the pastor visits, he could run the risk of bringing the disease into the congregation. Don't argue with the comments of any of the class members.

4. Jesus was not afraid to reach out and help the lepers. His love for us motivates us to follow His example and care for the sick among us, even if they have AIDS. In regard to the risk of contracting AIDS, within casual contact, there is little if any risk. Where exposure might exist, protective caps, gowns, gloves, and masks should be used.

Focusing on God's Word

(*About 15 Minutes*)

1. Have participants read 1 Corinthians 12:12–27 and underline the words or phrases that speak to the church about Peter and his family. When they are finished, encourage volunteers to share what they underlined.

(a) St. Paul describes the church as one body made up of many parts. We have all been baptized by the same Spirit, so we are the same body. Just as the eye can't say to the hand, "I don't need you!" neither can any member of the church say to Peter, "You're not one of us." Every Christian is an important, necessary part of the body of Christ. (b) It is fair in the sense that each part of the body is responsible for every other part. Peter is just as responsible for his neighbor as his neighbor is for him. (c) This seems unfair. But this is exactly what Jesus did. Jesus suffered and died for the sins of the whole world. By Jesus' death on the cross God provides forgiveness to repentant sinners.

2. Have participants read Matthew 25:31, 34–40, underlining words which they think describe Barbara's family. After doing so, have them pair off and share with each other what they underlined. When you bring the group back together, allow all the participants to brainstorm on how the Christian community could meet the Lord's expectations with reference to this family.

3. (a) When Peter returned home with AIDS, his family realized there were things about him they never knew, in effect making him a "stranger." Now, not only is Peter "sick," but the sickness is affecting his entire family. Peter and his family must often feel as though they are in "prison," serving an irrevocable sentence. (b) Christ is the head of the body, and all members of the body are one unit. In this way, whatever we do or don't do for one of our brothers or sisters is the same as if we do or don't do it for Jesus.

4. Jesus was filled with compassion. Remind participants that Jesus gave His life for us so that we might receive forgiveness of sins and eternal life.

5. We are all one in Christ, so, in a spiritual sense, if one has AIDS, we all share in it. But through the death and resurrection of Jesus Christ we have been made righteous and given the gift of eternal life.

6. God provides full and complete forgiveness through faith in Christ Jesus to all repentant sinners.

Focusing on My Life

(*About 10 Minutes*)

Have participants break into small groups to discuss questions 1 and 2. Then with the entire group read the paragraph detailing the four main ways that HIV is spread. Be sure to let participants know that the risk of contracting AIDS through casual contact is extremely low.

3. Let participants answer this question privately, allowing time for reflection.

4. Allow volunteers to share their personal experiences. Do not pressure anyone into sharing if they don't want to. Let participants brainstorm ways they or their congregation might effectively minister to people with AIDS or to families who are facing situations similar to Peter's parents.

Focusing on the Week Ahead

(*About 2 Minutes*)

Encourage participants to spend some time this week

studying information about the HIV virus and AIDS. Ask them to consider how they might use the information to better equip themselves and the people within their congregation to deal with the disease.

2

AIDS—Judgment or Grace?

❖ Focusing Our Sights

(*About 2 Minutes*)

Read aloud and discuss briefly the goals for this session.

❖ Focusing Our Attention

(*About 5 Minutes*)

Ask a volunteer to read aloud the second entry of "A Mother's Diary."

❖ Focusing on the Issue

(*About 10 Minutes*)

1. Returning home because he is too sick and weak to care for himself is a bittersweet experience for Peter—bitter because he has fulfilled his father's worst judgments about him and sweet because home will be a haven of care he so badly needs.

2. Remind participants that Peter's illness is a result of his actions, not God's judgment. Lack of judgment toward the person does not equal consent to sin. By judging others, we simply run the risk of hardening their hearts. Point out to participants that there is a difference between judging a person's sinful behavior as sin and judging the person. We must as Christians condemn sin, but demonstrate love to sinners. Through our sharing of God's Law—abhorrence for sin—and

God's Gospel—love for sinners through Jesus—the Holy Spirit works to call sinners to repentence.

3. Through sharing God's love for all people—sinners—the Holy Spirit leads people to repent and receive the assurance of God's love and forgiveness through Jesus.

4. When Jesus sat down with prostitutes and tax collectors to minister to them, He was not sanctioning their sinful acts. Instead, He was by His love demonstrating God's love for all people and desire that all people be saved.

5. When Peter is surrounded by caring Christians who are living the Gospel, the power of the Holy Spirit will work through them to call Peter to repentance and salvation. Then, even in death, Peter will be assured of eternal life with God.

Focusing on God's Word

(*About 15 Minutes*)

Have a volunteer read aloud John 9:1–5.

1. (a) According to the Scripture, a person afflicted with specific debilitating disease or illness does not necessarily indicate that the person or his/her parents were more sinful than anyone else. In some cases disease is a consequence of a person's sin, but in other cases it is simply a result of sin in the world. (b) In the cross God judges repentant sinners as "not guilty." Jesus came to save sinners from God's judgment toward us. In fact, Jesus took the judgment for sin upon Himself when He suffered and died on the cross. AIDS is a consequence of sin, not God's judgment on sin. (c) Jesus makes it clear that the man's sickness is not a punishment for his sin. However, sinful actions do have consequences: "A man reaps what he sows" (Galatians 6:7b). If Peter did indeed contract aids through illicit sexual behavior, then he is suffering the result of his actions. (d) Through Peter's illness, the work of God can be displayed in his life. Whether or not Peter is physically healed of AIDS, the greatest work of God would be Peter's call to faith in Jesus Christ through the power of the Holy Spirit.

Have a volunteer read aloud Luke 15:11–24. Have the participants break into small groups to answer questions 2 and 3. Allow a few minutes for discussion and then bring the group back together. Ask a representative from each group to share their answers. Remember that the key to the parable is that the father was filled with compassion for his son and gave him his love and forgiveness unconditionally, even though the son had done nothing to deserve it. The son approaches the father in repentance and the father graciously forgives. In the same way, God loves and forgives us because of His grace and compassion, not because of anything we've done.

Have a volunteer read Luke 15:1–2.

4. Jesus showed love and compassion for people who were considered the worst of sinners. He continues to shower His love and compassion on those we might consider the "chiefs of sinners," offering forgiveness and eternal life.

Have a volunteer read aloud Matthew 9:12.

5. Ask participants to read 2 Corinthians 5:17–20. Direct them to underline what Jesus did because of His love for sinners and His desire to treat their sickness. Next, have them circle the words which describe what God has now commissioned us to do, including for people who are dying of AIDS. When they are through, allow volunteers to share what they underlined and circled. Answers will vary. The life and death of Jesus reconciled the world to God—the issue now is the reconciliation of the individual to God by the power of the Holy Spirit working through the means of grace as we state in our confession of faith. This definitely includes those who are dying of AIDS.

❖ Focusing My Life

(*About 10 Minutes*)

1. Allow participants time to record their answers privately in their books.

2. Of the four choices given, *d* best describes forgiveness.

As God is moved with compassion and forgiveness, so we are led to compassion and forgiveness for others with our whole hearts, whether they are "deserving" or not.

3–4. Allow participants time to read and answer these questions on their own. Then invite them to share their responses.

❖ Focusing on the Week Ahead

(*About 2 Minutes*)

Encourage participants to spend some time in meditation and prayer in the next week, reading passages such as Matthew 18:21–35 and 1 John 4:7–13. Urge them to ask that God would help them care for those who might be infected with the HIV virus or AIDS.

3

AIDS—The Disease That Isolates

❖ Focusing Our Sights

(*About 2 Minutes*)

Read aloud and discuss briefly the goals for this session.

❖ Focusing Our Attention

(*About 5 Minutes*)

Ask a volunteer to read aloud the third and fourth entries of "A Mother's Diary."

❖ Focusing on the Issue

(*About 10 Minutes*)

1. Barbara, a "people person," feels separation from friends, the church, the neighborhood, and even God Himself. Sin always separates. It breaks relationships. God in His love sent Jesus to restore broken relationships with God and with others. Answers will vary.

2. Barbara is feeling isolated from her friends and her church family. This is partially because people sometimes back off when they are confronted with an unfamiliar situation. In the same way, the uncertainty of *What will they think? How will they treat us?* is keeping Barbara from reaching out to anyone.

3. Barbara writes that she had been praying for Peter

while he was gone. Now that he is back and dying of a terminal disease, Barbara is probably wondering if God heard her prayers at all. The hopelessness of the situation even makes reading her Bible seem purposelessness.

Focusing on God's Word

(*About 15 Minutes*)

1. In Genesis 2:18, 20–24, God has created woman to be man's helper. In Genesis 3:6–7, we find that the woman, after being tempted herself, tempts her husband, and they both sin against God. (a) In Genesis 2:18, God says "It is not good for man to be alone." God intended for people to be connected to each other. (b) Their eyes were opened, and they realized that they were naked. (See Genesis 3:7.) (c) A loving God could not bear to be separated from His people. Have a volunteer read aloud His solution in Romans 5:10.

2. Have a volunteer read aloud John 5:1–9. (a) Barbara feels totally isolated from anyone who could offer her support. She feels that she has no one. (b) The pool was surrounded by people who were too busy trying to see to their own needs rather than to help the man (v. 7). When no one showed him compassion, he must have felt very alone. (c) The man was cured of his paralysis as well his isolation apparently because Jesus wanted to show the healed man that He was the promised Savior and that even a greater healing was available—a healing of forgiveness and life eternal (v. 14).

3. Ask a volunteer to read aloud the words of David in Psalm 13:1–3. (a) The fact that even King David felt separated from God shows us that it can happen to anybody. David was a man after God's own heart, yet he also felt isolated at times. (b) The enemy in Barbara's life is the disease, fear, loneliness—anything which separates her from her one true Friend, God Almighty. Others can help Barbara see her real Friend, Jesus, by allowing God's love to be reflected through them.

❖ Focusing on My Life

(*About 10 Minutes*)

1. Allow participants time to answer this question on their own.

2–4. Have participants break into small groups to discuss these questions. Answers will vary. If time permits invite small groups to share their responses.

❖ Focusing on the Week Ahead

(*About 2 Minutes*)

Just as Barbara felt loneliness, so we feel lonely and isolated at times, even from God. Encourage participants to read the following passages from Scripture as a reminder to them of God's promises in loneliness: Psalm 23, Psalm 27:10, Psalm 42, Psalm 91:11, Isaiah 41:10, Matthew 28:20, Hebrews 13:5–6.

4

Healing from God

❖ Focusing Our Sights

(*About 2 Minutes*)

Read aloud and discuss briefly the goals for this session.

❖ Focusing Our Attention

(*About 5 Minutes*)

Ask a volunteer to read the fifth and sixth diary entries of "A Mother's Diary." Note the difference in Barbara's home in these two entries.

❖ Focusing on the Issue

(*About 10 Minutes*)

1. Barbara feels more connected because her friends and church family are reaching out to her and because she is allowing them to be a part of her experience.

2. Barbara feels connected with God again. Now that the wall of isolation is down, she is able to pray once more. Wes is getting along better with Peter, as they begin to respect each other. Remind participants that God provides the power to heal brokenness in His Word. Through God's Word the Holy Spirit works to create and strengthen faith.

3. John 13:35 says, "By this all men will know that you are My disciples, if you love one another." By loving and caring for Wes, Barbara, and Peter, the Christian community is giving the public an example of God's love in action.

4. Answers will vary. Contact by the Christian community will provide support and encouragement during Peter's last days on earth.

Focusing on God's Word

(*About 15 Minutes*)

Ask a volunteer to read aloud Luke 24:13–32.

1. (a) The disciples were supporting each other as they grieved the death of Jesus. Likewise, Barbara needs support as she prepares for the inevitable death of her own son. (b) In response, Jesus explained to the disciples everything that the Scriptures said about Himself. God provides faith-strengthening power to believers through His Word. (c) By reciting the Old Testament prophecies, Jesus was trying to assure His disciples that their grieving was unnecessary. He had risen, just as the prophecies foretold. (d) The text proves that Jesus was helpful because the disciples' hearts burned within them while He was speaking.

2. Jesus Christ was "perfectly broken" when He died on the cross. God's glory was revealed in His resurrection. The disciples were also broken in spirit over the happenings of the last week. Jesus, however, comes to them in their brokenness and gives them hope.

Ask a volunteer to read aloud Psalm 73:16–17a, 21–25.

3. Allow participants to reflect on this question. Remind them of the faith-strengthening power God offers through His Word.

Ask a volunteer to read aloud Colossians 3:13–14.

4. (a) Wes needed forgiveness for not treating his son as a loving father would treat his son. (b) Barbara needed forgiveness for cutting herself off from God and others. (c) Peter needed forgiveness for his lack of repentance and for his past lifestyle. (d) The congregation needed forgiveness for not supporting the family immediately. (e) The pastor needed forgiveness for letting Peter's past at first hinder him from ministering to Peter.

Share with participants that the message of the Gospel is one of forgiveness through Jesus Christ. We are all sinful people, but through Jesus Christ, we receive forgiveness.

❖ Focusing on My Life

(*About 10 Minutes*)

1. Allow participants time to read and answer this question on their own. Invite volunteers to share their responses.

2. Ask participants what they think of the quote by Mother Teresa. Answers will vary. Share with participants that God invites sinners to come to Him.

3. Ask volunteers to share how this study has increased their appreciation of the importance of the Christian community's support of individuals and families in crisis. Don't force anyone to share if he or she doesn't feel comfortable.

Ask a volunteer to read the seventh entry in "A Mother's Diary." God's grace has overwhelmed Barbara, Peter, Wes, the pastor, and the congregation. Only the Gospel can transform lives tainted by sin.

4. (a) After the funeral, Barbara will still need support as she grieves the death of her son. (b) Answers will vary. Some ways of supporting those who grieve the loss of a loved one include just being there, visits, listening, pastoral calls, prayer, and encouraging worship.

❖ Focusing on the Week Ahead

(*About 2 Minutes*)

Encourage participants to take time this week to reflect on how they and their congregation might help others in their struggle with AIDS or any other disease.